BEATING
BAD BREATH

Your Complete Guide To
Preventing and Eliminating Halitosis

Richard A. Miller, D.D.S.

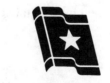

American Literary Press, Inc.
Baltimore, Md

BEATING BAD BREATH

Library of Congress
Cataloging in Publication Data
ISBN 1-56167-202-5

Published by

American Literary Press, Inc.
8019 Belair Road, Suite 10
Baltimore, Maryland 21236

Manufactured in the United States of America

" According to a former chief rabbi of Israel, bad breath is a legitimate reason for divorce. Schlomo Goren was quoted by the Item News Agency as saying several couples were granted divorces in recent years after citing halitosis . . . "

newspaper article

CONTENTS

A Short Sad Story

The evening is coming to a close and Mark is beginning to feel a bit nervous. He's had a nice time with Susan, but will she kiss him good night?

"Thanks for a nice evening, Mark," Susan says.

"I had a good time, too. May I kiss you good night?"

Smiling, she nods her approval.

Slowly Mark moves his head toward Susan. Quicker than the blink of an eye, her nose catches the odor of bad breath. She turns her head and his kiss lands on her cheek.

Embarrassed, Mark turns and runs down the stairs.

An imperfect end to an otherwise perfect first date.

Do You Have Halitosis?

Are you one of the millions of people who suffer from halitosis, or bad breath?

If you do have halitosis, you're not alone.

It has been estimated that 56-65% of the population has chronic bad breath. What's more, according to *Geriatrics*, a prominent medical journal, halitosis gets worse as we get older. In fact, halitosis is so widespread, that *over $500 million is spent every year to cover it up with mouthwashes, sprays, and breath mints.*

What's even more astonishing is that if you have halitosis, *you probably don't even know it!* And don't expect your friends or family to tell you—that's just not done. What they'll do instead is shy away from you or kiss you on the cheek—anything to get away from your breath.

Test Yourself For Halitosis

Try this simple test:

Take a piece of white, unflavored dental floss (thick) and use it between 4 upper and 4 lower *back* teeth. Move the floss around for a few seconds in each place, then look at it. Is it discolored? Wait a moment. Smell the floss. Is there an odor?

Still not sure? Try this.

Take a piece of clean gauze—it's available at any drugstore. Stick your tongue out and, firmly, wipe the furthermost back portion of your tongue two or three times. Wait a moment, then smell the gauze. Is there an odor?

If either of these tests is positive, it's a good bet you have halitosis.

Note: It's important when doing either of these tests to wait a moment before smelling the floss or gauze. Why? The same reason that we have a hard time detecting our own bad breath.

It's called *adaptation*—a sensory phenomenon peculiar to taste and smell. Have you ever entered a room with a particularly bad odor? After you stay in the room awhile the odor seems to get better. In reality the odor is still there, but you have "adapted" to it: lost your awareness of it. So it is with our own halitosis. It's also why people in close proximity to us, and even our loved ones, may at first smell our bad breath, but then seem not to notice it as their own protective adaptation comes into play.

Current Treatment Is Not Effective

Americans spend over *500 million dollars* annually for fresher breath. Why? Because up until now, the only treatment for halitosis has been to cover up a bad odor with a stronger, more pleasant-smelling one. Not only does this do nothing for the cause, it's not even very effective!

In 1992, *Consumer Reports* tested the efficacy of 15 mouthwashes that claimed to eliminate bad breath. Their tests found that while all the mouthwashes tested were still working 10 minutes after being used, only *some* were working after one hour—and those only partially. *Consumer Reports* concluded "...the results varied too greatly from person to person to generalize; no product proved to be consistently better than any other...at the end of two hours, they all had fairly little residual effect."

$500 million for products that don't work very well.

What Does All This Mean To You?

Plenty.

If, that is, you'd like never to worry about bad breath again.

In this book we'll acquaint you with the causes of halitosis. We'll note the latest research and tell you what works and what doesn't. And we'll give you a program to follow no matter what your oral condition may be.

In short, we'll tell you how to keep your breath fresh and kissably sweet.

PART I

THE PROBLEM:

WHY WE GET BAD BREATH

What Causes Bad Breath?

Contrary to popular belief, our breath is not influenced by what is happening in our stomach. In other words, an "upset stomach" or an "acid stomach" does not affect our breath. That's because air from our upper gastrointestinal tract does not mix with the air we exhale, unless we have esophageal reflux or hiatal hernia.

In fact, medical problems are behind only a very small percentage of bad breath cases even though conditions such as sinusitis, emphysema, and diabetes can sometimes cause bad breath. In some cases, bad breath can also be attributed to medications such as decongestants and antihistamines, but this too, is infrequent. (For a more complete listing of medical conditions and drugs see Appendix B.)

It is important to note that the medical causes for halitosis represent less than 10% of the total.

The plain fact is, while there are some medical reasons for bad breath, the *overwhelming cause of halitosis comes from what happens in our mouths.* Even offending foods and tobacco cause only a small percentage of bad breath problems.

Before we look at the oral causes, let's examine two other reasons for halitosis—offensive foods and tobacco.

Offending Foods

We've all had the experience of eating our favorite foods only to end up with bad breath as a result. (My wife never hesitates to tell me when I smell like garlic or onions. I guess a plumber's wife is quick to complain about a leaking faucet.)

Bad breath from foods starts when the membranes of our mouth and throat absorb some of these odors. The resulting odor can last a few hours; some foods, like garlic and onions result in odors that are even longer lasting.

When these foods are digested, small odor molecules get into our bloodstream, some finding their way to our lungs. Mixed with air, we exhale these odor molecules causing bad breath. Many foods besides garlic and onions, like radishes, cabbage, and cauliflower can have this effect. In fact, garlic is so powerful that garlic odor on the breath can be detected after garlic is rubbed on the feet!

Before any important social or business situation, it may be wise to avoid these odor-causing foods—even though the treatment recommended later will help alleviate the odors caused by them. And, keep in mind that, compared to the 90% of halitosis with oral causes, this is still a small part of the problem.

Tobacco

Having come into contact with people who routinely smoke cigarettes or cigars most of us are familiar with smoker's breath. Many people who smoke, even though they're usually unable to detect their own odor are aware that their habit causes a type of halitosis. Remember adaptation? This phenomenon is particularly evident in smokers who have been smoking for some time.

The odor from tobacco occurs for two reasons. Primarily responsible is the accumulation of tar, nicotine, and other noxious substances on the tongue, cheeks, teeth, and other tissues of the mouth. You may have noticed this accumulation as a brownish-black stain on the teeth. However, a lesser known reason—and one that contributes to the long-term nature of the halitosis in smokers is the drying effect that tobacco has on the membranes of the mouth. (More on this drying effect later.)

Obviously, the best way to eliminate this bad odor is to stop smoking. We're all aware that doing that benefits our lungs and overall health as well as our breath. But if you're not ready to stop smoking, there are still effective ways to rid yourself of tell-tale breath, as we'll see in Part III.

Oral Causes

By far the overwhelming cause of halitosis is oral. Here's how it happens.

The mouth is, of course, the home to numerous bacteria. Some of these bacteria are responsible for dental decay; some for gum disease; and some for various mouth infections. These same bacteria are also responsible for halitosis.

The odors of halitosis come from bacterial production of *sulphur compounds*—from the proteins we eat, from debris, and from the cells of the mouth lining that are shed in a natural process like the outer layer of our skin. Not unlike the production of body odor by bacteria under our arm, these sulphur compounds, if left untreated, create the odor of halitosis. You're probably familiar with one type of these sulphur compounds—hydrogen sulfide—the same compound that causes the smell of rotten eggs.

The bacteria that cause halitosis are from a family of bacteria termed "anaerobic." Unlike "aerobic" which means "with air," these bacteria thrive in places where there is little or no air—under the gums, in the crevices of the tongue and between the teeth—where they multiply and create halitosis. And they are especially active in gingivitis and gum disease and on the surface of the tongue.

These bacteria also thrive when the environment of the mouth gets out of balance as in the case of "morning breath."

Morning Breath

We don't sense it, but our mouth harbors a *slightly* acid environment. Our saliva, among its many important functions, serves to balance the acid level of the mouth making it an unfriendly place for bacteria. When this slightly acid level gets weak or disappears, the halitosis-causing bacteria thrive. In fact, this is the primary cause of "morning breath."

When we sleep, because our saliva flow diminishes, certain areas of the mouth become fertile breeding grounds for bacteria and the production of sulphur compounds. Even if we sleep with our mouth open, the air we inhale through our mouth, along with the lessened saliva, dries our mouth lining, allowing bacteria deep under the gums and in the crevices of our mouth to flourish and create the same sulphur compounds.

The key here is the diminished flow of saliva. In fact, *as we age, saliva flow naturally decreases, resulting in an increase in halitosis.*

Gingivitis & Gum Disease

Gingivitis is the name given to inflammation of the gums. *Gum disease* or *periodontal disease*, usually a progression of gingivitis, results when the bone under the gum becomes destroyed.

Gingivitis occurs when dental plaque—a residue of food, bacteria, and acids—accumulates around the teeth and is not adequately removed. This provides a fertile environment for the production of halitosis. In some cases, the gums become inflamed, tender, swollen, and even bleed on occasion when brushed or flossed. (Contrary to what some people believe, occasional bleeding of the gums is *not* normal.)

As more plaque accumulates, the deeper layers harden forming tartar which creates a breeding ground for live bacteria. This makes removal of the bacterial laden plaque under the gum even more difficult and gum disease begins. As gum disease progresses, these deposits cause the gums to pull away from the teeth and the bone to dissolve creating gum pockets and allowing more bacteria to accumulate at an even deeper level on the tooth root—a vicious cycle. Amazingly enough, this process is mostly painless!

While these bacteria are destroying bone and causing the gum disease to progress, they are also producing the sulphur compounds that cause halitosis. Hidden under the gums these bacteria flourish making the gums the #1 site for production of halitosis.

How Do You Know If You Have Gum Disease?

Unfortunately, gum disease is usually silent, causing few noticeable symptoms. Since these symptoms are usually painless many people ignore the warning signs. The principle warning signs of gum disease are:

1. Gums that bleed when you brush or floss.

2. Red, swollen, or tender gums.

3. Gums pulled away from the teeth.

4. Pus around the teeth and gums.

5. Loose teeth.

6. Change in bite or tooth position.

7. Bad taste or bad breath.

Please note that you cannot self-diagnose gum disease. In many cases, even X-rays taken on a regular basis will not show beginning or sometimes even moderate loss of bone. The only way to determine if gum disease is present is to ask a dentist to perform a gum exam.

In a gum exam, the dentist measures the space between the gum and tooth. Since healthy gums are tightly attached to the tooth, a separation of more than 3 millimeters (approximately 1/8 inch) indicates gum detachment and gum disease. The higher the reading, the greater the problem. (See diagrams following page)

Gum Exam and Gum Disease

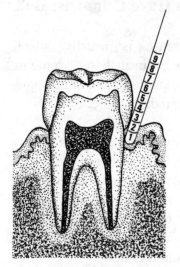

Healthy Gums
Measures 3mm or Less*

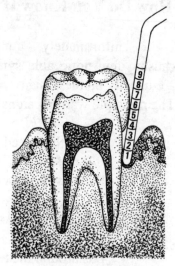

Early Gum Disease
Measures 4-5mm*

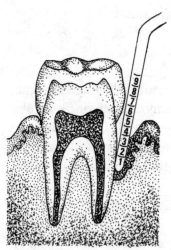

Moderate Gum Disease
Measures 6-7mm*

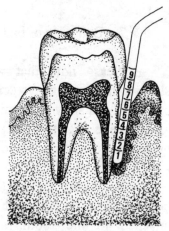

Severe Gum Disease
Measures 8mm or More*

*Factors other than pocket depth are also important in classifying gum disease.

The Tongue

The second most common site of halitosis-causing bacteria is the tongue, where they usually go undetected, protected by the many coatings that cover the tongue's surface.

If one were to examine the tongue with a magnifying glass, one would see small and large projections, like different-shaped mushrooms, arising from its surface. These "papillae" contain our taste buds, different ones for different tastes—sweet, sour, salty, and bitter. It is among these projections that bacteria flourish in a warm, low-air environment and produce the sulphur compounds of halitosis.

The tongue coatings, which protect the bacteria, come from many sources, especially thick food substances left behind after swallowing. Foods like milk, thick juices, creamy foods, sauces, even stain-causing foods like coffee and tea leave behind substances that lodge in the papillae and cover the bacteria, allowing them to grow undisturbed. In order to eliminate halitosis, we must remove the tongue coating to get to these bacteria.

Other Breeding Grounds

Dentures, Partials, and Other Appliances

Dentures, partial dentures (removable bridgework), and other mouth appliances are also breeding grounds for halitosis causing bacteria. Since the plastics which make up these prostheses are porous, bacteria lodge in the imperfections and, nourished by food that gets under the appliance, create halitosis. And if you add the penetrating ability of the sulphur compounds to the porosity of the plastic it is easy to see why dentures themselves oftentimes have an odor.

Faulty Dental Work

Another problem area is faulty dental work. Ill-fitting fillings or restorations can contribute to halitosis by promoting the accumulation of bacteria and food particles which in turn promotes the formation of sulphur compounds. In fact, any place where food gets trapped—between the teeth, under bridgework, or under fillings—is a breeding site for halitosis causing bacteria.

Moved, Drifted or Extruded Teeth

When missing teeth are not replaced, the stability of the mouth is jeopardized as the remaining teeth shift to try to fill the space. When this occurs, new spaces open up where food and bacteria can accumulate which, in turn, creates breeding grounds for the bacteria which produce sulphur compounds and halitosis by the fermentation of the trapped food particles.

16

Dental and Gum Abscesses

Tooth and gum abscesses are the end stages of decay and gum disease, respectively. While there may be warning signs along the way, even pain, some abscesses perforate the bone and gum tissue allowing sufficient drainage as to not be painful. Called fistulas, these infectious drainage sites can go on for some time without closing, constantly draining pus into the mouth with its resultant bad taste and putrid mouth odor.

Other Causes

There are other oral conditions which contribute to halitosis that are worth mentioning.

Oral thrush (candidiasis) is common in older adults and occurs when the bacteria of the mouth are overridden by a yeast-type organism in people who are chronically ill or who are taking medications such as cortisone drugs or antibiotics. The odor caused by candidiasis is usually not the sour odor of halitosis, but a sweeter, fruity-type odor.

Oral cancer represents 2.5% of all cancers in women and 5% of all cancers in men. While the odors caused by long-standing oral cancers may mimic that of halitosis, there is also the odor of dead tissue present. Please be aware that the use of this taste and smell to self-diagnose cancer is ill advised due to the process of adaptation described previously. If any unusual sores, lumps, or bumps appear, they should be checked by a dentist.

SUMMARY

90% of halitosis comes from oral causes.

Halitosis is especially prevalent in gum disease.

Medical conditions constitute a small part of halitosis.

Food and tobacco contribute to halitosis but are not a primary cause.

Halitosis is caused by *sulphur compounds*.

Sulphur compounds are produced by bacteria that live in the mouth.

The primary sites for these halitosis-causing bacteria are the gums and tongue.

Other mouth conditions related to halitosis are:
    wearing dentures or partial dentures
    faulty dental fillings
    drifted, moved, extruded teeth
    gum or tooth abscesses
    oral thrush or oral cancer

PART II

THE SOCIAL DILEMMA:

DO YOU TELL SOMEONE THEY HAVE BAD BREATH?

How Do You Break The Bad Breath News?

Perhaps you didn't just pick up this book for yourself. Perhaps your real motivation is the bad breath of a friend, a business associate, or a loved one. Now that you know how to determine if *you* have bad breath, how do you tell someone close to you?

How you tell someone that he or she has halitosis will depend on a variety of factors. To begin with, ask yourself:

How well do you know this person?
What is our relationship?
When would be the best time? The best place?
When would it be especially important?

The approach you use depends on the relationship you have with this person. While this chapter will offer you a number of suggestions, only you can determine the best way to approach the subject of bad breath.

Here's how Tom did it.

The interview was only a week away and Mary was getting nervous. She was applying for a new job and wanted everything to be perfect. She had purchased a new suit and was to have her hair done on Saturday. But she had some concerns about her breath, especially since she hadn't had her teeth cleaned in 3 years.

"Tom, do I have a problem with my breath?" she asked her husband.

"Well, honey," Tom replied sheepishly not quite sure what to say, "I have noticed an odor occasionally."

Mary decided to see for herself and ran some floss between her back teeth—sour.

"Tom, you're right. What should I do? My big interview is in less than a week."

"Mary, there may be a solution. A friend at work told me about a similar problem he had. His dentist cleaned his teeth and gave him some special mouthwash and in 2-3 days, his breath was back to normal. Why don't you give him a call?"

Mary did just that. After a dental cleaning and the use of a new mouthrinse and toothpaste she got from her dentist, her breath was fine by Sunday.

And she got the job!

Here Are A Few Suggestions

1. To begin with, it's important to be as gentle and sincere as possible. In discussing this problem with someone you care about, start by being careful about the word you use to describe bad breath. It would be wise to use words like "sour" or "strong" rather than "offensive."

2. Remember, halitosis is simply a condition—one that can be temporary—not a defining characteristic. That means it can be changed, and as we shall see, fairly easily.

3. By telling someone, you can assume the role of helper, not detractor.

4. One method that may prove effective is the matter-of-fact approach.

a. Suggestion: "Honey, I thought this book looked interesting so I picked it up at the bookstore today. Tell me what you think."

b. Suggestion: "Joe, I found this book useful so I picked up an extra copy. Here. Let me know if you agree."

5. In other circumstances, the best approach may be a direct one:

a. Suggestion: You know your colleague is facing an upcoming important meeting, yet his breath is offensive. You could say, "Joe, this is a time you may want to pay special attention to your breath." Then give him a copy of this book.

b. Suggestion: You're about to become intimate with someone, yet their breath is a turn-off. Be honest now. "Honey, this is a time you might want your breath to be especially pleasing."

In either case, if you use the direct approach you'll want to have on hand some of the products mentioned later to offer concrete help to your colleague or loved one.

6. Sometimes, the best way to deal with a serious subject is with humor.

a. Suggestion: Gift wrap this book without a card and leave it on someone's desk.

b. Suggestion: Slip this book into your spouse's briefcase or into a drawer at home.

One reason that people don't tell others about their bad breath is that, until now, there was little to be done about it. As a mentor of mine once said, "There's nothing worse than bad breath covered by a hint of mint."

7. Because, as you'll see in the next chapter, there are simple and effective ways to eliminate bad breath at its source, not just cover it up, you might want to try an optimistic tactic.

a. Suggestion: "You know, Joe, there's something I've thought of mentioning for some time. But until now, I didn't have any good suggestions. Now, I do. This book may be just the thing."

8. One of the best ways to tell someone about his or her bad breath is by the use of a relevant anecdote. Your little story can be real or hypothetical.

      a. Suggestion: "I thought you might like to know, I once had a friend who had a particularly bad problem with strong breath. So bad, in fact, that her career went nowhere. But when she discovered she could treat it, her confidence soared and her career took off."

While it's true that some of these methods demand a bit of courage, remember that if you notice someone's bad breath, others do too. In fact, bad breath may be having a negative effect on this person's life, one which they may not even be aware.

So, do the halitosis sufferers in your life a favor. No matter how you decide to go about it, let them know they have bad breath.

PART III

THE SOLUTION:

HOW WE CAN GET RID OF
BAD BREATH

Proper Oral Care Eliminates Halitosis

The evidence is overwhelming: *To end—or prevent—halitosis, you must eliminate the bacteria in your mouth and the sulphur compounds they create.*

Wait, I know what you're going to say: "My dentist already has me brushing after meals, flossing twice a day, using baking soda and stimulating my gums. It's taking over my life! What I want is a simple way to keep my mouth fresh and get rid of bad breath forever."

Well, you're in luck. Simplicity is here. New technology and new techniques can help you eliminate halitosis and improve your oral hygiene in just a few minutes twice a day.

We're going to show you which techniques work best and how to implement them in an easy-care program *that really works*. And, equally important, we'll introduce you to some new oral care products that are producing amazing results!

But don't forget your dentist. Because of the relationship between gum disease and halitosis, as well as the many other oral causes, you'll want to make him or her an important part of your team as we'll show you in Part IV.

The Tools

The Toothbrush

For centuries, the toothbrush has been the primary method for removal of bacteria and food from the teeth, gums, and other mouth areas. Early toothbrushes were constructed from plant stalks and leaves, while brushes in later years were made from animal hair, much like shaving brushes. Today, toothbrushes are mass produced with different shapes, sizes, heights, lengths, and even thicknesses of bristles. The best brushes are soft and engineered to be the same diameter as the average gum space around the tooth for easy removal of bacteria.

Proper hand brushing can be very time consuming taking at least five minutes twice a day.

Enter technology.

A few years ago, the electric toothbrush took a turn for the better with the advent of rotational toothbrushes. With multiple heads rotating together, these brushes allowed the same sideways brushing motion that people use with their hand brushes to reach many more nooks and crannies where bacteria hide. The amount of time spent in any given area could be reduced thanks to the rotating bristles. However, too vigorous use of these could damage the gums.

The Ultimate Toothbrush

But electric toothbrushes shared one inherent flaw with hand brushes—they still needed to touch all the tooth and gum surfaces to be effective. Yet any gum pocket, even small ones, were usually out of reach of these brushes. With the recent development of ultrasonic toothbrushes, this is no longer as critical. Using this type of toothbrush, a person does not have to be a clockmaker to develop a precision technique for oral care.

An ultrasonic toothbrush merges ultrasound technology into the head of a toothbrush to create a vibration. These ultrasonic waves emitted from the brush head—and carried by toothpaste, saliva, and other fluids in the mouth—can dislodge the bacteria under the gums. In this way, they disrupt the destructive process and halitosis production.

When used with a similar but slower brushing technique as you would a hand toothbrush, an ultrasonic toothbrush can lead the fight against halitosis causing bacteria.

Flossing

As your dentist has no doubt told you, using only a toothbrush for the removal of bacteria is not enough. There are numerous places a brush cannot reach, even an ultrasonic brush. To complement toothbrushing, dental floss was invented.

You say you don't like to floss?

Two new advances in dental floss have made this unpopular activity easier:

1. Dental floss coated with Teflon has reduced the difficulty of manual flossing by making the up and down movements of the floss easier.

2. The most innovative breakthrough: the ultrasonic flosser. Whereas in conventional flossing, a large degree of dexterity is necessary to hold the floss in the many different angles necessary to do an adequate job, the ultrasonic flosser does the work for you. It takes the frustration out of dental flossing.

When combined with an ultrasonic toothbrush, the ultrasonic flosser creates the best combination available for at-home halitosis elimination.

Irrigators

One of the latest tools to make a big splash in the dental home care market has been the water irrigator. Ranging from pulsating jet sprays like those in showers to pinpoint water jets, these devices promised to remove almost everything a toothbrush couldn't reach—and the advertising worked. But in actuality, on the lower settings, they aren't strong enough to remove the bacteria; and on higher settings, they can potentially harm the gums.

However, these devices do have an important use in cases of gum disease. The technique involves a blunt-ended needle that allows you to irrigate the deepest gum pockets. This needle, called a "cannula" should only be used under the care of a dentist for it requires a degree of dexterity and practice to avoid injury.

While most irrigators simply direct a stream of plain water onto the teeth and gums, a recent innovation shows a great deal of promise. Termed a hydromagnetic irrigator, it uses the same principal as industry does to remove deposits in a moisture-filled environment. These hydromagnetic irrigators use a magnetic field to ionize the water particles which then work more effectively against sticky bacteria-laden plaque and tartar deposits. While not the final answer, when used with the proper anti-bacterial solution (p. 41), the hydromagnetic irrigator becomes a valuable addition to the home care techniques for eliminating halitosis.

Tongue Scraper

One final device must be mentioned for halitosis care—the tongue scraper. While this is not a device recommended by many dentists, because it does nothing for the teeth and gums, and while most drugstores have never heard of it, it is one of the most valuable tools against halitosis.

Earlier I pointed out that the tongue, particularly the backmost part, was the second largest site for bacteria and sulphur compounds. The easiest and most comfortable way to remove the many layers of tongue coatings that hide these bacteria is the tongue scraper.

A tongue scraper is simple to use. Just stick your tongue out, place the curved portion as far back on the tongue as you can and pull forward with a moderate, scraping pressure. While this is a routine that only takes a few seconds to perform, it's a valuable addition in the fight against halitosis.

Mouthwashes

Over the centuries, many different oils and potions have been used to cover up bad breath, and today is no exception. Just as perfumes can cover body odors, mouthwashes simply use a stronger odor to cover up the existing halitosis. However, this technique which is used by virtually every mouthwash on the market doesn't really work.

As already mentioned, *Consumer Reports* rated a number of over-the-counter mouthwashes and found that while all covered up the odor being tasted (garlic) for ten minutes, a smaller number were still working after one hour, demonstrating their lack of staying power. (Best to do all your kissing in the first 10 minutes.) Is it not a coincidence that the same companies that manufacture mouth rinses also manufacture breath sprays—a convenient method to continually cover up mouth odor when the mouthwash dissipates?

However, a potentially greater problem with over-the-counter mouthwashes is their alcohol content. Alcohol, a common household disinfectant, has been used to kill germs on surfaces for years. In fact, nurses rub it on our arms before giving a shot or taking blood. While it is somewhat effective against the bacteria that inhabit the mouth, its major drawback is that alcohol has a drying effect on the mouth tissues. You may recall that one of the contributing factors to halitosis is dryness of the mouth! *So these products provide short-term relief while creating a long-term problem.*

Aside from their lack of lasting effectiveness and their drying effect on the mouth tissues, there is also some question regarding safety of some mouthwashes. A 1991 study performed at the National Cancer Institute and quoted in the *Journal of the American Dental Association* indicated that mouthwashes "containing more that 25% alcohol could increase the risk of oral and pharyngeal cancers by about 50%."[1]

The alcohol contents for some mouthwashes are listed below:

Listerine	26.9%
Scope	18.9%
Cepacol	14%
Plax	8.5%

Is it worth the risk?

Toothpaste

A brief word on toothpaste is in order. Like mouthwashes, toothpastes contain substances that cover up the odors of halitosis, but do not eliminate them. While some are recommended for sensitive teeth, some for freshening breath, and others for tartar control, none is effective in eliminating the bacteria or destroying the sulphur compounds of halitosis.

---

[1] JADA 1993;124:55-64

CLO$_2$

By far the greatest advance in halitosis management has been the formulation of mouthwashes and toothpastes that are effective against sulphur compounds. Unlike conventional products, those containing CLO$_2$ (pronounced "C," "L," "O," "2") actually *destroy the sulphur compounds at the molecular level.* That's right, *destroy, not cover up.*

CLO$_2$, otherwise known as chlorine dioxide, has been used in water purification for over fifty years and has been certified safe by the Environmental Protection Agency. CLO$_2$ in mouthwashes and toothpastes is totally safe for use in the mouth and solves many of the problems inherent in over-the-counter mouthwashes and toothpastes.

Here's what they do:

1. **Maximum Effectiveness**

    One of the problems inherent in halitosis is that the bacteria that create sulphur compounds are most active when the environment of the mouth is out of balance. CLO$_2$ products are manufactured to be active in a slightly acid environment which restores this balance and reduces bacterial activity. This slightly acid environment is highly effective against bacteria, but is *not* harmful to the mouth.

2. **Safe**

Unlike conventional mouthwashes, there is absolutely no alcohol present in CLO_2 products, so there are no worries about increased risk of cancer.

3. **Works Microscopically**

By now it should be no secret that the mouthwash you are currently using is not very effective because it simply covers up odors. CLO_2 breaks the molecular bonds that give sulphur compounds their odor. In other words *CLO_2 works at the source— destroying odor, not covering it up.*

4. **Long Lasting**

CLO_2 products have been shown to be effective for *5 hours* after use.

5. **Helps Gum Disease**

Since gum disease is caused by bacteria you might expect that any substance that reduces bacteria would help gum disease. Until now, however, you have had to put up with the trade-offs of potentially cancer-causing alcohol and a very low level of effectiveness. Enter CLO_2. By actually destroying the sulphur compounds, CLO_2

helps to inhibit the penetration of bacteria into the gums.

In fact, the research on CLO_2 has uncovered even more benefits. In a recent study it was shown that the use of a CLO_2 mouthwash and a CLO_2 toothpaste would actually *reduce the size of the gum pockets!* In the study, 1,406 gum pockets out of 2,085, or 67.4%, were healed to a depth of less than 3 millimeters, the optimal depth for gum health.[1]

That's not all! There's other important research about CLO_2.

An article published in the February 1995 issue of the dental journal *Compendium* showed the positive effect of CLO_2 on gum bleeding. You may recall that bleeding gums are not normal and almost always signal gum disease. In fact, when a gum exam is performed, the presence of bleeding is a conventional indicator for gum disease. In this article, in a total of 639 gum pockets with bleeding, 71.8% showed no bleeding after 6 months when CLO_2 was used in a mouthwash and toothpaste twice a day.[2] And this was without any dental treatment!

It is readily apparent that CLO_2 is the most effective means for controlling halitosis and, according to the research, it can even help gum disease. When combined with a proper oral care program, CLO_2 will not only freshen your breath but also improve the health of your mouth!

---

[1] Compend Cont Ed Dent 1994;15(6):740-46
[2] Compend Cont Ed Dent 1995;16(2):188-96

Want even more evidence? Try this:

The Onion Test

Take a raw onion and cut a slice no greater than one-eighth inch. Immerse it in a CLO_2 mouthwash for a minimum of two minutes (the amount of time you would normally rinse). Remove the onion and smell it.

The odor is completely gone, isn't it?

Note: If the onion slice is greater than one-eighth inch, the CLO_2 will need a longer time to penetrate the onion. If it is too thick, the CLO_2 will not get to the inner core. In this respect, the onion is different from your mouth, where the swishing action when you rinse would deliver the mouthwash to every area of the mouth.

Or, try this:

The Garlic Test

Rub a wet cotton swab onto some garlic. Then dip the same swab into a small container of CLO_2 mouthwash for one minute. Smell the swab.

Don't smell anything, do you?

Benefits Of CLO_2

Eliminates halitosis
Non-toxic
Reduces gum bleeding
Reduces some gum pockets
Non-alcoholic
Non-carcinogenic
Environmentally friendly
Low abrasion (toothpaste)
Kills bacteria

By now you should be convinced that CLO_2 is without a doubt the safest and most effective substance against the sulphur compounds that cause halitosis.

Where can you get CLO_2?

Mouthwashes and toothpastes, as well as other CLO_2 products, are available through your dentist.

However, to eliminate the plaque that harbors the bacteria of halitosis, gum disease, and decay, CLO_2 must be combined with a proper oral hygiene regimen.

Here then, is the

No-Nonsense Halitosis Elimination Program.

The No-Nonsense
Halitosis Elimination Program

Rinse with CLO_2 mouthwash AM and PM. Rinse two minutes or more each time. Rinse more frequently if you have eaten odor-causing foods.

Brush with CLO_2-containing toothpaste AM and PM. Brush your teeth and gums for at least two minutes, using an ultrasonic or rotational toothbrush.

Wipe your tongue with a gauze, being sure to wipe the backmost portion or, better yet, use a tongue scraper to remove the outer coating. Then brush your tongue with a CLO_2 toothpaste and a hand or rotary toothbrush for 1 minute or until the tongue looks pink.

Floss with an ultrasonic flosser (or by hand) at least once daily.

If halitosis is a persistent problem, feel free to rinse with a CLO_2 mouthwash more frequently.

If you wear dentures, use the following regimen.

Rinse with CLO_2 mouthwash AM and PM. Rinse for two minutes or more each time.

Wipe your tongue with a gauze or tongue scraper. Brush your tongue as well as the roof of your mouth with a CLO_2 toothpaste. A rotary brush can be used on the tongue, but do not use it on the delicate gum areas.

Wipe your gum areas with a gauze then rewipe with a gauze that has CLO_2 toothpaste on it.

Brush your dentures with CLO_2 toothpaste in the morning and evening.

Soak your dentures in CLO_2 mouthwash at night.

You may also use a tongue scraper after meals as well as the CLO_2 mouth rinse as the need arises.

If you wear other mouth appliances:

Follow the first program as explained above, however, also brush your appliance with CLO_2 toothpaste and soak your appliance at night in a CLO_2 mouth rinse. (If your dentist advises not removing the appliance at night, soak it for an hour or two during the day in a CLO_2 mouthrinse.)

If you smoke:

Follow the basic regimen, however, to maintain halitosis-free breath you should increase the frequency of rinsing with CLO_2 and brushing with CLO_2.

Rinse with CLO_2 mouthwash AM and PM. Rinse two minutes or more each time. If possible, rinse with a CLO_2 mouthrinse after smoking.

Brush with CLO_2-containing toothpaste AM and PM. Brush your teeth and gums for at least two minutes, using an ultrasonic or rotational toothbrush.

Wipe your tongue with a gauze, being sure to wipe the backmost portion or, better yet, use a tongue scraper to remove the outer coating. Then brush your tongue with a CLO_2 toothpaste and a hand or rotary toothbrush for 1 minute or until the tongue looks pink.

Floss with an ultrasonic flosser (or by hand) at least once daily.

The use of a plain gauze to wipe the tongue and cheek areas after smoking and the periodic use of a tongue scraper will eliminate a large number of sulphur compounds and the tar and nicotine that coat the tongue.

Because smoking dries out the mouth, you may want to try a "saliva substitute." These substances stimulate your saliva glands to produce more saliva and, unlike commercial gums and mints, are buffered for the optimal mouth environment.

**If you have a medical condition that causes halitosis
or if you take mouth-drying medications:**

Follow the basic regimen using CLO_2 mouthwash and toothpaste twice each day for a minimum of two minutes each time.

Be sure to use an ultrasonic toothbrush and ultrasonic flosser for best plaque removal.

Use a tongue scraper or gauze regularly to remove tongue coatings.

Ask your doctor about using a saliva substitute to moisten the mouth and inhibit the growth of bacteria. This also helps in gum disease and decay prevention.

PART IV

THE PROFESSIONAL APPROACH

Remember the sad story of Mark and Susan's first date?

Well, here's:

A Happier Ending

Mark was devastated by Susan's rejection. He had known Susan for six months before he got up the courage to ask her out. And now, after their first date, he doubted he'd get another. In his mind's eye, he kept seeing himself kissing her cheek instead of her lips. Finally, it dawned on him. "Maybe its my breath" he thought.

He decided to check it out. The next morning, he took a piece of gauze from his medicine chest and wiped his tongue. Yellow. Then he smelled the gauze. Sour.

At work that day, Mark cornered his best friend.

"Rick, tell me the truth. Do I have a problem with my breath?"

Rick nodded. "Afraid so. I've noticed it more than once. If you're interested, I may have a solution. Call my dentist."

Mark called and got some professional help. Using CLO_2 mouthrinse and toothpaste supplied by his new dentist, his breath improved. In a week, it was no longer a problem.

Mark celebrated by sending Susan a dozen roses with a note: "Problem solved. How about Saturday night?"

The rest, as they say, is history.

Professional Diagnosis & Treatment

While the at-home halitosis treatments that we've already detailed are highly effective, because of the link between gum disease and bad breath, as well as the other mouth problems that can contribute to bad breath, it may be wise to seek the help of a dentist to diagnose and treat halitosis.

The dentist who diagnoses and treats halitosis must be familiar with the following:

> medical causes of halitosis
> instruments for measuring halitosis
> correct halitosis treatment

Let's examine these in greater detail.

Dental Exam For Halitosis

A dental exam for halitosis must start with an understanding on the part of the dentist of the many illnesses and medications that can cause bad breath. Before examining your mouth, a dentist familiar with halitosis would thoroughly review your past and current medical history, past dental treatment, at-home care, and oral health history. Only with a thorough interview, can the dentist uncover any hidden causes of halitosis.

After the interview is complete, the actual dental exam should take place. To diagnose and treat halitosis properly, your dentist will use an instrument called a Halimeter, which scientifically measures the volume of sulphur compounds in the breath. Another invaluable instrument in halitosis diagnosis and follow-up is the Periotemp, an instrument that measures inflammation in the gum spaces. While halitosis is intimately related to gum disease, the bacteria that cause both problems start their work in the gum space—with inflammation as a result. The Periotemp measures the temperature differential between healthy and inflamed gum areas and is a valuable tool in detecting the sources of halitosis as well as the activity of gum disease. As it measures bacterial activity, it also allows the dentist to measure the level of bone loss.

For proper halitosis diagnosis, these diagnostic instruments must be combined with X-rays and a complete visual examination, since hidden causes such as tooth infections and yeast can only be uncovered in this way.

Professional Treatment

When your dentist has completed the examination for halitosis, the treatment phase can begin. To treat halitosis properly, a dentist must individualize treatment in the following areas:

1.   **In-Office Bacterial Control**

This is the essence of professional halitosis treatment, and involves the removal of bacteria from under the gums where they colonize and create sulphur compounds. In some cases this may involve simple cleaning procedures; however, in the case of gum disease, further treatment may be indicated.

2. **Gum Disease Treatment**

Remember, the gums are the primary site for halitosis causing bacteria. Even with the use of CLO_2 products, a dentist or dental hygienist must remove the odor causing bacteria that have accumulated under the gums.

3. **At-Home Care**

To be effective, in-office bacterial control must be combined with proper at-home care. It is important when personalizing treatment that the dentist be familiar with the different oral hygiene tools available so as to guarantee proper bacterial control.

4. **Proper Maintenance**

With professional treatment, monitoring the level of halitosis is an integral part of the process. Using the Halimeter and Periotemp, the dentist can follow your progress and be able to make any necessary modifications.

With professional treatment, your dentist can find the hidden causes of halitosis and improve the health of your mouth.

QUESTIONS ABOUT HALITOSIS

Q: If halitosis is caused by bacteria, why not take antibiotics to kill them?

A: No antibiotic regimen can kill all the bacteria in our mouths. While a strong dose of antibiotics would reduce the bacterial population for a time, it increases the risk for other problems—sensitivity, overgrowth of yeast, immunity, etc.

Q: Is there a test for halitosis?

A: Yes, there is. Some dentists can test for mouth odor with an instrument called a Halimeter that measures the level of sulphur compounds. Other tests that measure the number of bacteria and the type of bacteria are also available. Two invaluable tools that we use are a microscope to view the relative activity of the bacteria, and a Periotemp that measures the degree of bacterial activity in the gum pockets.

Q: Does stained teeth mean I have halitosis?

A: Not necessarily. It depends on the amount of stain and how long it's been there. The best way to determine if you have halitosis is by trying the two tests at the beginning of this book or asking your dentist to test you for it.

Q: What should I do if I suspect gum disease?

A: The first thing to do is get a gum exam. Most moderate and some advanced cases of gum disease can be treated without surgery. In fact, new research shows that a non-surgical technique is just as successful as surgery in many cases. Some general dentists are now specially trained in nonsurgical gum treatment.

Q: What if my child has bad breath?

A: If you are concerned about a baby or infant, I would suspect a medical problem—milk allergy, or colic, most likely. See your pediatrician. For older children, I recommend just checking their diet. Diets high in sugars will allow the sulphur-producing bacteria to flourish. If you're satisfied that the diet is okay, next check their oral hygiene. Since gum disease is not likely, seeing a dentist is your best bet.

Q: Do sensitive teeth indicate gum disease?

A: Many times, yes. The only way to find out is to ask your dentist to perform a gum exam. If he or she does not do a gum exam routinely, find one who does. Remember, even X-rays do not show many cases of early and moderate bone loss.

Appendix A

CLO$_2$ PRODUCTS

<u>Oxyfresh, USA</u>
Oxyfresh™ mouthwash
Oxyfresh™ toothpaste
Oxyfresh™ Gel
Oxyfresh™ Deodorizer

<u>Rowpar Pharmaceuticals, Inc.</u>
Retardex™ (mouthwash)
Retardent™ (toothpaste)

ULTRASONIC TOOTHBRUSH
Ultra Sonex®

ULTRASONIC FLOSSER
Floss Plus® Easy Flosser

HYDROMAGNETIC IRRIGATOR
Hydro Floss®

SALIVA SUBSTITUTE
Salix™

Appendix B

Some Possible Medical Causes of Halitosis	Some Possible Drug Causes of Halitosis
RESPIRATORY	
sinusitis	DMSO
tuberculosis	amyl nitrate
emphysema	chloral hydrate
tonsillitis	paraldehyde
tumors	metronidazole
pharyngitis	antidepressants
pneumonia	antiparkinsonians
bronchitis	antipsychotics
	narcotics
LIVER	decongestants
liver failure	antihistamines
liver cirrhosis	antihypertensives
gall bladder disease	anticholinergics
KIDNEY	
uremia	
GASTROINTESTINAL	
esophageal reflux	
hiatus hernia	
stomach cancer	
malabsorbtion	
SYSTEMIC	
diabetes	

BIBLIOGRAPHY

Braun RE, Cianco SG. Subgingival delivery by an oral irrigation device. *J Periodontol* 1992; 63:469-72.

Bosy A, Kulkarni GV, Rosenberg M, *et al.* Relationship of oral malodor to periodontitis: evidence of independence in discrete populations. *J Periodontol* 1994;65(1):37-46.

Chapek CW, Reed OK, Ratcliff PA. Reduction of bleeding on probing by oral care products. *Compend Cont Ed Dent.* 1995;16(2):188-96.

Chapek CW, Reed OK, Ratcliff PA. Management of periodontitis with oral-care products. *Compend Cont Ed Dent* 1994;15(6):740-46.

Claycomb CK, Schearer TR. Malodors of the Mouth. *J Oreg Dent Assoc* Summer 1986:34-35.

Durham TM, Malloy T, Hodges ED. Halitosis: 'Knowing when "bad breath" signals systemic disease. *Geriatrics* 1993;48(8) August: 55-59.

Johnson BE. Halitosis, or the meaning of bad breath. *J Gen Int Med* 1992:7:649-56.

Kleinberg I, Westbay G. Salivary and metabolic factors involved in oral malodor formation. *J Periodontol* 1992; 63(9): 768-75.

Krause KK, Graham GS, Stoffers KW, Dennis MA. The effectiveness of chlorine dioxide in the barrier system. Presented at the 1989 Thomas P. Hinman Meeting, Atlanta, GA.

McDowell JD, Kassebaum DK. Diagnosing and treating halitosis. *JADA* 1993:124:55-64.

O'Heihir T. Ugh! What can we do about that awful morning mouth? *RDH* 1992 Apr;12(4):12.

Ratcliff P, Bolin V. Antimicrobial Capacity of chlorine dioxide based toothpaste. Presented at IADR meeting, 1993.

Ratcliff P, Bolin V. ClO_2/phosphate germicide vs. Actinobacillus Actinomycetemcomitans and Prophyromonas (bacteroides) gingivalis. Presented at the AADR meeting, 1992.

Ratcliff PA, Bolin V. Germicidal effect of povodine-iodide and CL02 on dental pathogens. Presented at AADR meeting, 1987.

Rosenberg M. First International Workship on Oral Malodor. *J Dent Res* 1994;73(3):586-89.

Rosenberg M, Kulkarni GV, Bosy A, *et al*. Reproducibility and sensitivity of oral malodor measurements with a portable sulphide monitor. *J Dent Res* 1991; 70(11):1436-40.

Rosenberg M. Bad breath: Diagnosis and treatment.*UTDJ* 3(2):7-11.

Rosenberg M, Septon I, Eli I, *et al*. Halitosis measurement by an industrial sulphide monitor. *J Periodontol* 1001;6298): 487-9.

Scully C, Porter S, Greenamn J. What to do about halitosis. *BMJ* Jan 22, 1994;308:217-18.

Terezhalmay GT, Gagliari VB, Rybicki LA, *et al*. Clinical evaluation of the efficacy and safety of the Ultrasonex ultrasonic toothbrush: A 30-day study. *Compend Contin Ed Dent* 1994;15(7):866-74.

Tessier JF, Kulkarni GV. Bad Breath:Etiology, diagnosis, and treatment. *Oral Health* 1991 October:19-24.

Touyz LZ. Oral malodor - a review. *J Can Dent Assoc* 1993;59(7):607-10.

Watt DL, Rosenfolder C, Sutton CD. The effect of oral irrigation with a magnetic water treatment device on plaque and calculus. *Jnl Clin Perio* 1003;20;314-17.

Yaegaki K, Sanada K. Volatile sulphur compounds in mouth air from clinically healthy subjects and patients of periodontal disease. *J Perio Res* 1992;27:233-8.

Yaegaki K, Sanada K. Biochemical and clinical factors influencing oral malodor in periodontal patients. *J Periodontol* 1992;63(9):783-9